Copyright 2023

Table of Contents

PREVIEW

An inflammation or infection in one or more small pouches in the digestive tract.

Diverticulitis is more common after the age of 40.

Symptoms include abdominal pain, fever, nausea and a change in bowel habits.

Treatment can include rest, a liquid or low-fibre diet and antibiotics. Severe cases may need hospital care and surgery. Doctors may recommend a high-fibre diet after recovery to prevent future episodes.

Diverticulosis is a medical condition when small, bulging pouches form on the wall of your bowel. On the other hand, diverticulitis is the medical condition when those pouches get inflamed or infected. Together, these two conditions are known as diverticular disease.

Although it was rare before the 20th century, diverticular disease is a very common health problem in the Western world. It's a group of conditions that can affect your digestive tract.

The most serious type of diverticular disease is diverticulitis. It can cause uncomfortable symptoms and, in some cases, serious complications. If left untreated, these complications can cause long-term health problems.

Both sexes are equally affected by diverticular disease and diverticulitis, although the condition is more likely to appear at a younger age (under 50) in men than in women. Overall, symptoms of diverticulitis are most likely to occur in people over 70 years old.

People aged 50-70 who eat a high-fibre diet (25g a day) have a 40% lower chance of admission to hospital with complications of diverticular disease – compared to others in their age range with the lowest amount of dietary fibre.

Fiber helps to soften stools, and not consuming enough dietary fiber leads to hard stools. This may cause more pressure or strain on the colon as muscles push the stool down. This pressure is thought to cause the development of diverticula.

In parts of the world where dietary fiber intake is large, such as in Africa or South Asia, diverticula disease is fairly uncommon. On the other hand, it is quite common in Western countries where dietary fiber intake is much lower.

DIVERTICULITIS DIET RECIPES

BREAKFAST

1. Savory Quinoa Bowls

Prep Time: 5 Minutes

Cook Time: 25 Minutes

Servings: 4

Ingredients

- 1 medium sweet potato, peeled, cubed (large dices)

Extra-virgin olive oil, for drizzling

- ½ teaspoon seasoning of choice (salt/pepper, etc.)
- 2 cups – 2 ½ cups cooked quinoa (⅔ – ¾ cup uncooked) – adjust amount as desired
- ⅔ – 1 cup chickpeas, drained and rinsed
- ½ – ⅔ cups cherry tomatoes, chopped
- 1 avocado (medium), peeled and diced
- 2 scallions, finely chopped, green portion only
- 1 handful spinach leaves (optional)

Protein & Toppings/Garnishes

- Olive oil or dressing of choice

- Juice of ½ lemon, to taste
- Sea salt to taste
- Ground black pepper to taste
- 3– 4 hard-boiled eggs, sliced or eggs in olive oil
- ⅓ Cup parsley, chopped

Instructions

1. Preheat the oven to 400°F, and line or grease a baking sheet.
2. Toss the sweet potatoes with a drizzle of olive oil and a few pinches of seasoning of choice. Roast 20-25 minutes or until they are tender and golden.
3. In a large bowl, toss the roasted sweet potatoes with the cooked quinoa, chickpeas, tomatoes, avocado, scallions, and optional spinach.
4. Drizzle the ingredients with olive oil (or a dressing of choice), lemon juice, and salt and pepper to taste. Toss and serve into bowls or meal prep containers.
5. Top each bowl with a sliced hard-boiled egg or one fried egg.
6. Garnish the bowls with fresh herbs and seasoning to taste.

7. Meal Prep/ Make-Ahead Tip: To save time, prepare the bowl ingredients a day before (minus the avocado). Divide the ingredients into meal prep containers or mason jars. Add the avocado, olive oil, lemon, and remaining toppings right before serving or taking on the go.

2. Air Fryer Sausage (Gluten Free)

Prep Time: 5 Minutes

Cook Time: 15 Minutes

Servings: 12

Ingredients

- 1 ½ pounds ground sausage – chicken, turkey, or lean pork (pre-seasoned country sausage may be substituted, adjust spices below if so)
- 3 teaspoons minced garlic
- 1 teaspoon crushed red pepper flakes
- 2 teaspoons fresh thyme leaves (or ½ teaspoon dried thyme)
- 1 teaspoon onion powder
- ½ teaspoon smoked paprika
- ¼ teaspoon cayenne
- ¼ teaspoon or to taste kosher salt
- ¼ teaspoons or to taste black pepper
- Optional: 2 sage leaves, chopped
- 2 teaspoons maple syrup, honey, or raw sugar

Instructions

1. In a large bowl, combine the ground sausage and herbs and spices (garlic, chili flakes, thyme, onion powder, smoked paprika, cayenne, salt and pepper, and sage leaves), and sugar. Using two hands, mix the ingredients together until they are well-blended.

2. Shape the sausage mixtures into patties about 3 to 3 ½ inches wide and 1 to 1 ½ inches thick.

3. Place the formed patties on a baking tray lined with parchment paper to keep them from sticking.

4. Spray the air fryer basket with cooking oil. Preheat the air fryer to 375 degrees Fahrenheit.

5. Once preheated, place 4-5 patties in the air fryer.

6. Air fry the sausage patties 12-15 minutes on manual, flipping halfway through cooking. Check for doneness at 10-12 minutes.

7. Remove the sausage patties from the air fryer, place them on a clean plate, and cover them to keep warm. Repeat the steps above, air frying the remaining patties.

8. Serve with sauce of choice.

3. Green Chile Egg Casserole

Prep Time: 10 Minutes

Cook Time: 40 Minutes

Servings: 8

Ingredients

- 2 hatch green chile pepper
- 1 teaspoon olive oil or avocado oil
- 1 cup baby spinach
- 1 cup chopped white onion
- 10 –12 eggs (12 eggs for a denser texture)
- 1 cup nondairy milk
- 3 Tablespoon tapioca flour or cornstarch
- 1 teaspoon baking powder
- ½ teaspoon salt
- ¼ teaspoon pepper
- ½ teaspoon cumin
- Pinch of garlic powder
- 1 teaspoon minced garlic
- 8 ounces (or two 4 ounce cans) chopped green chiles, drained

- 6 ounces sliced cheese (parmesan, mozzarella, white cheddar)
- 1 plum tomato, sliced
- Grated hard cheese for topping (optional)
- Fresh chopped cilantro

Instructions

1. Preheat the broiler. Line a baking sheet with foil.
2. Place the Hatch green chile pepper on the foil. Once the broiler is ready place the peppers in the oven, and broil them for 3-4 minutes on each side or until the skin is browned. Remove the peppers from the oven, and set them aside.
3. Turn the oven temperature down to 350 degrees Fahrenheit.
4. In a small pan, add 1 teaspoon of oil, and sauté the onion and spinach together on medium to medium high heat for about 3 minutes or until they are fragrant. Remove the pan from the heat.
5. In a large bowl, beat the eggs and milk on medium-high speed with an electric mixer until they are light and fluffy. Add the flour (or starch), baking powder, salt, garlic powder, pepper, and cumin.

6. Blend the ingredients for about 30 seconds until they are just combined and smooth. Stir in the canned green chilies (8 ounces).

7. Layer the bottom of an 8×11 casserole dish with the cooked spinach and onion. (See notes for other sizes of dishes.)

8. Then, add a few slices of cheese, followed by the egg and green chile batter.

9. Once cooled, peel the skin off the roasted hatch green chiles and slice them length-wise, removing the stem. Layer the top of the casserole with tomato, slices, sliced roasted Hatch green chiles, and more cheese.

10. Place the casserole in the oven, and bake for 30-40 minutes. Check the casserole after 30 minutes. If the outside is brown but the inside is still not set, cover the dish, and continue to bake for an additional 5 to 10 minutes. For crispy edges, set the oven to broil the last minute of cooking.

11. Remove the casserole from the oven. Sprinkle it with extra cheese (if desired) and fresh cilantro. Season to taste.

4. Vegan Mushroom Bacon Toast (Gluten Free)

Prep Time: 5 Minutes

Cook Time: 30 Minutes

Servings: 5

Ingredients

For the Smoky Vegan Bacon (Mushroom Bacon)

- 1 ¼ cup or 6 ounces finely diced or chopped mushrooms (shiitake or oyster mushrooms work best). For quick crispier mushroom bacon, use dried mushrooms.
- Olive oil to drizzle
- Kosher salt and pepper to taste
- ½ tsp smoked paprika and/or 1 tsp liquid smoke
- ⅛ Tsp onion powder or garlic powder (or pinch of both!)
- 1 tsp coconut sugar or maple syrup

For the breakfast toast –

- 4–5 pieces Gluten free whole grain bread –
- ½ c + plain hummus or garlic hummus (Sabra)
- Grape or cherry tomatoes

- Chopped Herbs (fresh parsley or basil to top)
- Kosher salt and pepper
- Olive oil to drizzle
- Other Optional toppings –
- Nutritional yeast "for Cheesy" taste
- Large sea salt flakes or smoked sea salt flakes
- Crushed red pepper flakes
- Cracked black pepper or peppercorns

Instructions

1. FIRST: See instructions for making toast to save time on meal prep in the oven!

For the smoky mushroom vegan bacon:

2. Preheat oven to 375 F. Line a baking sheet with parchment paper, or well-oiled the sheet pan.
3. Finely chop the mushrooms into smaller pieces and place on sheet in a single layer. Drizzle 1 teaspoon olive oil on top of mushrooms and season with kosher salt and optional pepper.
4. Place mushroom in the oven and bake for 12- 15 minutes. After 12- 15 minutes, remove from the oven and toss or carefully flip mushrooms over. Return

mushrooms to the oven and continue cooking until browned and crispy, about 12-15 minutes.

5. Remove from the oven. Place mushrooms in a bowl or plate and blot the oil off. Then toss with coconut sugar or maple syrup, garlic and/or onion powder, smoked paprika, and optional liquid smoke. Return mushroom back to the pan and in the oven to caramelize. About 5 minutes longer.

6. Remove and set aside for breakfast toast topping.

7. Make your breakfast toast –

8. Before returning the mushrooms to the oven the second time, prep the sheet pan with your toast and tomatoes. Oil the pan and place toast on top and tomatoes in a foil pack or on another pan. The toast and the tomatoes pan will be placed on top or bottom rack. All can cook in the oven at the same time I like to place the toast and tomatoes in a separate pan and bake with the last 10 minutes. The tomatoes will blister and soften. The toast will brown.

9. After the toast and mushrooms are ready, layer your ingredients.

10. Spread 2 tablespoons of hummus on each piece of toast, then add a few blistered tomatoes, followed by

vegan mushroom bacon bits, herbs, and cracked pepper, sea salt.

11. Repeat for each piece of toast.

5. Healing Porridge

Prep Time: 9 Minutes

Cook Time: 11 Minutes

Servings: 2

Ingredients

- 2 to 3 Tablespoons lightly toasted sunflower seeds or 1 Tablespoon tahini
- 2 Tablespoons unsweetened shredded coconut
- 1 Tablespoon chia seed or flaxseed (omit for AIP or substitute with 1 Tablespoon collagen/gelatin powder)
- 1 teaspoon ground ginger
- ½ teaspoon ground cinnamon
- Pinch ground turmeric
- Pinch kosher salt
- ½ cup water or coconut milk, more if needed
- 1 cup chopped and cooked butternut squash, kabocha or acorn squash
- Pure maple syrup or raw honey
- If using Instant pot you will need additional coconut oil or ghee and water

- Toppings – berries, cherries, pomegranate seeds, coconut cream or coconut yogurt

Instructions

1. In a blender, add sunflower seeds, shredded coconut, chia seeds, ginger, cinnamon, turmeric and salt. Blend until the mixture is a flour-like consistency. If short on time, use tahini instead of sunflower seeds, and mix the ingredients together in a bowl until smooth. (No blender required).

Stove Top Instructions

2. In a small bowl, add the dry mixture with water or coconut milk, stirring to combine. Set aside to thicken. Feel free to save a little bit of the gel for topping!
3. Add the cooked squash and sunflower seed mixture into a blender, and blend until smooth.
4. Heat the mixture in a saucepan on the stove top over medium heat for 5 minutes or until it starts to bubble, stirring occasionally.
5. Remove from the heat and divide into bowl(s). Optional – To help improve digestion and absorb more nutrients stir in 1 teaspoon ghee.

6. Top with optional toppings, and serve immediately while warm.

Instant Pot Instructions

1. Peel and chop the squash into large pieces. Place in the Instant Pot with ½ – 1 Tablespoon coconut oil. Sprinkle with cinnamon and nutmeg (or cloves) and SAUTE for 5 minutes, turning the squash a few times.
2. Add ⅓ cup water to the cooking pot. Lock the Instant Pot lid and set the vent to close. Select MANUAL mode and cook on high pressure for 5-6 minutes.
3. Allow a natural pressure release or use a quick release if short on time. Unlock the lid, and carefully drain the hot water. Add in the dry mixture of blended seeds/spices and a splash of non-dairy milk and puree with a hand blender.
4. Serve immediately or place the lid back on and keep it on WARM mode until ready to serve. Top with optional toppings.

6. Bread Pudding with Pecan Crumble Topping

Prep Time: 2hrs 2 Minutes

Cook Time: 60 Minutes

Servings: 6

Ingredients

For the bread pudding:

- Unsalted butter (about 1/2 tablespoon), for greasing the pan
- 1 pound brioche bread, cut into 3/4-inch cubes
- 8 eggs
- 2 cups milk
- 1/2 cup heavy cream
- 1/2 cup sugar
- 1/2 cup packed light brown sugar
- 1 tablespoon vanilla extract
- 2 tablespoons good bourbon
- Pinch of fine grain sea salt
- 1/2 cup chopped pecans, toasted

For the crumble topping:

- 1/2 cup flour

- 1/2 cup chopped pecans
- 1/2 cup packed dark brown sugar
- 1 teaspoon cinnamon
- 1/4 teaspoon fine grain sea salt
- 3 tablespoons unsalted butter, at room temperature
- Sliced persimmons, for serving
- Maple syrup, for serving

Instructions

1. Lightly butter a 9-by-13 baking dish, then place cubes of brioche in the baking dish in an even layer.

2. In a large bowl, whisk together eggs, milk, heavy cream, sugars, vanilla, bourbon and a pinch of sea salt. Sprinkle toasted pecans over the brioche, then pour the custard evenly all over the bread. Gently press the bread down into the liquid. Cover and let sit in the fridge for at least 2 hours (or up to overnight).

3. Once you are ready to bake the bread pudding, take the baking dish out of the fridge and preheat an oven to 350°F. Meanwhile, prepare the crumble. Add flour, pecans dark brown sugar, cinnamon, salt and butter to a medium bowl, and using your fingertips, rub

ingredients together until evenly combined and clumps start to form. Sprinkle the surface of the bread evenly with the crumbs. Bake until the bread pudding is puffy and the top is golden (45 minutes to an hour). Let cool for a few moments before serving.

4. To serve, cut squares of warm bread pudding, and place on small plates. Top with sliced persimmons and maple syrup. Enjoy immediately!

7. Carrot Cake Chia Pudding

Prep Time: 15 Minutes

Cook Time: 00 Minutes

Servings: 1

Ingredients

- 1 cup unsweetened almond milk
- 1 Medjool date, pitted
- 1/2 teaspoon ground cinnamon
- 1/4 teaspoon ground cardamom
- 1/4 teaspoon ground ginger
- Pinch of grated nutmeg
- Small pinch of sea salt
- 1/4 teaspoon vanilla extract
- 3 tablespoons chia seeds
- 1/2 cup grated carrot, from 1 large peeled carrot
- 1 tablespoon chopped walnuts

Instructions

1. Add almond milk, dates, cinnamon, cardamom, ginger, nutmeg, salt and vanilla to a blender, and blend until

smooth. Place chia seeds in a medium bowl, and pour over spiced almond milk, stirring to combine. Cover and chill in the fridge for at least 15 minutes (or up to 3 days). Stir 3 times during the first 15 minutes to break up any clumps of chia seeds.

2. To serve, stir in grated carrot and walnuts.

8. Chorizo and Spinach Scramble

Prep Time: 35 Minutes

Cook Time: 11 Minutes

Servings: 1

Ingredients

- 3.5 ounces about 1 red skinned potatoes, diced
- 1 tablespoons olive oil, plus more for drizzling
- 1/8 teaspoon cumin seeds, ground cumin will also work here, just use a little less
- 1/8 teaspoon paprika
- Sea salt
- Freshly ground black pepper
- 2 eggs
- 1 tablespoon unsweetened almond milk
- 2 tablespoons finely chopped onion
- 3 ounces high-quality fresh chorizo 2 ounces (about 2 handfuls) baby spinach leaves
- Fresh salsa, for serving
- Cilantro leaves, for serving (optional)

Instructions

1. Preheat an oven to 400°F.

2. Place potatoes on parchment-lined baking sheet, then toss with a drizzle of olive oil, cumin seeds and paprika. Season well with salt and pepper. Bake until tender, but not falling apart (30 - 35 minutes), stirring occasionally.

3. During the last 10 minutes of cooking, prepare the scramble. Whisk eggs and almond milk together in a small bowl. Warm 1 tablespoon olive oil in a medium skillet over medium heat, then add onion and cook until soft, but not brown (about 2 minutes). Next, add the chorizo to the skillet, and cook, stirring to break the pork into pieces, until brown and crumbly (3 - 4 minutes). Stir in the spinach, and cook, stirring frequently, until just wilted (about 2 minutes). Finally, pour in the eggs, and cook, stirring frequently, until scrambled and just set (2 - 3 minutes). Season to taste with salt and pepper.

4. To serve, spoon potatoes into a shallow bowl, then top with chorizo scramble. Finish with a few spoonfuls of fresh salsa and a scattering of cilantro leaves.

9. Candied Jalapeños

Prep Time: 5 Minutes

Cook Time: 10 Minutes

Servings: 20

Ingredients

- 1 cup apple cider vinegar
- 3 cups sugar
- 1/4 teaspoon cumin seeds
- 1/4 teaspoon celery seeds
- 1 1/2 teaspoons granulated garlic
- 1/2 teaspoon cayenne pepper
- 1 1/2 pounds jalapeños, stems removed, thinly sliced

Instructions

1. Add vinegar, sugar, cumin seeds, celery seeds, garlic and cayenne to a large pot, and bring to a boil over medium-high heat. Reduce to medium-low, and simmer for 5 minutes. Stir in the jalapeño slices, return to a simmer and cook for 4 minutes. Using a slotted

spoon, transfer the slices to a clean jar (I used a 28.7 oz weck jar).

2. Turn the heat up to medium-high and bring the remaining syrup to a rolling boil. Boil hard for 6 minutes. Using a ladle, carefully pour the boiling syrup over the jalapeño slices. The syrup should fully cover the slices (you'll have a little leftover). Insert a clean chopstick or skewer to the bottom of the jar two or three times to release any trapped air pockets. Cover the jar, and let cool completely before storing in the refrigerator. The candied jalapeños can be enjoyed immediately, but they're better if you let them mellow for 1 week to 1 month before eating.

10. Butternut Squash, Sausage and Parsnip Hash

Prep Time: 5 Minutes

Cook Time: 25 Minutes

Servings: 4

Ingredients

- 3/4 pound peeled butternut squash, cut into 1/2-inch dice
- 1/2 pound peeled parsnip, cut into 1/2-inch dice
- 4 tablespoons olive oil, divided
- 1/2 pound chicken and apple sausage
- Sea salt
- 1/2 small onion, chopped
- 2 garlic cloves, chopped
- Freshly ground black pepper
- 6 ounces about 1/2 bunch kale, stems removed, leaves sliced thin
- 2 teaspoons apple cider vinegar
- Torn parsley leaves, for serving

Instructions

1. Place chopped squash and parsnip in an even layer on a microwave safe plate, and cook on high in the microwave until heated through, but still firm to the touch (5 minutes).

2. Add 1 tablespoon oil to a large cast-iron (or non-stick) skillet, and warm over medium heat. Cook the sausage, stirring occasionally, until browned and fully cooked through (about 5 minutes). Transfer sausage to a plate and set aside. Wipe the skillet clean.

3. Return the skillet to a medium-high heat, warm 2 tablespoons olive oil and add the squash and parsnips along with a pinch of salt. Cook, stirring occasionally, until golden on most sides (4 to 5 minutes). You'll want to let the veggies cook undisturbed for 1 - 2 minutes, then toss, stir and repeat. Avoid moving the veggies around in the pan.

4. Add the onion to the skillet, season with salt and pepper, and cook, stirring occasionally, until tender (about 3 minutes). Stir in the garlic and cook until fragrant (30 seconds). Move the veggies to one half of the skillet. Place remaining tablespoon of oil in the other half of the skillet. Let the oil warm for a moment, then add the sliced kale and a small pinch of salt,

stirring to combine. Cook, stirring occasionally, until the greens wilt (2 to 3 minutes). Take the skillet off the heat, stir in the vinegar, and season to taste with additional salt and pepper. Stir in the cooked sausage, and let warm for a moment in the hot skillet.

5. To serve, spoon 1/4 of the hash in a shallow bowl and top with a scattering of torn parsley leaves. Store additional portions covered in the fridge.

LUNCH

11. Garden Grape Focaccia

Prep Time: 15 Minutes

Cook Time: 30 Minutes

Servings: 10

Ingredients

- 2 1/4 teaspoons active dry yeast (I used SAF yeast)
- 2 teaspoons honey
- 2 1/2 cups lukewarm water (between 95°F and 105°F)
- 5 cups (625 grams) all-purpose flour
- 5 teaspoons kosher salt (I used diamond crystal kosher salt here)
- 5 to 6 tablespoons extra virgin olive oil
- Unsalted butter, for greasing the pan
- Flaky sea salt, for topping
- Garden Toppings: halved red California seedless grapes, sliced red chiles, rosemary needles, Italian parsley leaves

Instructions

1. Add yeast, honey and water to a medium bowl, whisking to combine. Let sit for 5 minutes. Add flour and salt, then mix using a rubber spatula until a shaggy dough forms. Pour 4 tablespoons olive oil in a large bowl, then scrape the dough into the center of the bowl. Cover and let rest in the fridge for 24 hours.

2. Generously butter a baking sheet, then brush 1 tablespoon olive oil around the pan. Keeping the dough in the bowl, fold the furthest edge of the dough to the center. Turn the bowl 1/4 and then fold the next edge to the center. Repeat this 2 more times (so 4 folds total). Flip the dough over in the bowl (so the seam side is down), then transfer to the center of the prepared baking sheet (don't stretch it at this point). Pour any excess oil over the dough. Let the dough rise, uncovered, until doubled in size (2 to 3 hours). While the dough is rising a second time, prepare any toppings (halve the grapes, pick the rosemary needles, pick the parsley leaves, slice the chiles).

3. Preheat an oven to 450°F and place a rack in the middle setting. Lightly oil your hands and dimple the focaccia all over using your fingertips. If the dough has not expanded to the edges of the baking sheet, coax it to the

edges while you are dimpling. Sprinkle the top evenly with sea salt.

4. To decorate, arrange grapes, chiles and herbs on the surface of the focaccia. You don't want to place too many grapes in a cluster, because they'll weigh down the dough too much. Also, make sure any leaves are sticking to the surface (if not they'll burn). You don't want to cover the entire surface, so make sure you leave some areas blank. Work carefully and quickly while doing this. Drizzle a little olive oil over any of the blank spots (where just the dough is showing).

5. Bake until the focaccia is puffed and golden (20 – 30 minutes). Transfer to a cooling rack and let sit for 5 minutes. This focaccia is best enjoyed warm on the day you bake it (depending on toppings). Wrap any leftovers in parchment and store at room temperature for up to 3 days. Toppings like kale leaves and herbs will get soft over time, so warm up the focaccia in an oven before serving.

12. Instant Pot Carnitas

Prep Time: 5 Minutes

Cook Time: 55 Minutes

Servings: 8

Ingredients

- 2 teaspoons kosher salt (I used Mortons here), plus more to taste
- 1 1/2 teaspoons dried Mexican oregano, rubbed between your fingers to break into smaller bits
- 1 1/2 teaspoons ground coriander
- 1 1/2 teaspoons ground cumin
- 1 1/2 teaspoons freshly ground black pepper
- 4 1/2 pounds boneless pork shoulder, cut into 2" pieces
- 3 jalapeños, halved lengthwise
- 6 garlic cloves, peeled but left whole
- Zest of 1 orange
- Juice of 1 orange

Instructions

1. Add salt, oregano, coriander and cumin to a small bowl, stirring to combine.

2. Place about half of the pork in the bottom of an Instant Pot and season each piece with the spice mixture. Scatter half of the jalapeños, garlic cloves and orange zest on top. Top with remaining pork, then season those pieces with the remaining spice mixture (you'll use all of it). Top with remaining jalapeños, garlic cloves and orange zest. Pour orange juice down the side of the Instant Pot, so it reaches the bottom of the pot without disturbing all the spices.

3. Seal the lid and cook on high pressure for 45 minutes. Release the pressure manually, and using a slotted spoon, transfer pork to a large container. Shred meat using two forks, then season to taste with salt. Transfer cooking liquid to a fat separator, then pour some of the liquid back over the meat. You want to moisten the meat, but it shouldn't be covered or drowning in the liquids.

4. Working in batches, transfer the carnitas to large nonstick skillet set over high heat*. Cook, undisturbed until the bottom develops a golden crust (5 to 7 minutes). I like to brown just 1 side, so you get that

golden flavor without drying the pork out too much. At this point, the carnitas is ready for tacos, nachos, burritos or bowls.

13. Jorge's Green Chilaquiles

Prep Time: 10 Minutes

Cook Time: 25 Minutes

Servings: 6

Ingredients

- 1 1/2 pounds tomatillos (about 12 to 14), husks removed, rinsed and dried
- 1/4 onion
- 4 garlic cloves
- 1/4 cup packed cilantro leaves
- Kosher salt
- 1 tablespoon vegetable oil
- 1 cooked chicken breast, shredded
- 13 ounces freshly fried tortilla chips or thick cut store-bought tortilla chips
- 1 can (7.6-ounces) full fat media crema (or use heavy cream or sour cream thinned with a bit of water to pourable consistency)
- 8 ounces Oaxacan cheese, shredded (you can also use low moisture mozzarella here)

Instructions

1. Add tomatillos to a large skillet over medium-high heat, and cook, shaking the pan occasionally, until charred in spots and juices start to release (10 – 11 minutes). Transfer tomatillos to a blender along with the onion, garlic, cilantro, 2 tablespoons water and a few pinches of salt, and blend until smooth.

2. Warm 1 tablespoon oil in a small saucepan over medium heat, then add the salsa. Bring to a boil, reduce heat to low, and cook, stirring occasionally for 10 minutes. Season to taste with additional salt (flavors should be bold).

3. To assemble, place half the chips in a 12-inch skillet (preferably one with a lid!) in an even layer. Top with half of the shredded chicken, then 1 cup salsa. Drizzle Media Crema evenly over top, then sprinkle with a pinch of salt. Repeat the layers again, topping with remaining chips, chicken and 1 cup salsa (you'll have a little salsa leftover). Finish with an even layer of cheese.

4. Cover the pan and place over medium-low heat, and cook just until the cheese melts and the chips and salsa warm through (about 10 to 15 minutes). Serve immediately.

14. Smoked Curried Chicken Salad

Prep Time: 2hrs 2 Minutes

Cook Time: 6 Minutes

Servings: 4

Ingredients

- 2 pounds bone-in, skin-on chicken thighs (about 4 large thighs)
- Kosher salt
- Freshly ground black pepper
- 1 tablespoon + 2/3 cup olive oil, divided
- 1/2 yellow onion, diced
- 1 garlic clove, minced
- 2 1/2 tablespoons minced fresh ginger
- 1 teaspoon curry powder
- 1/2 teaspoon ground cumin
- 1/2 teaspoon ground turmeric
- 1/3 cup white vinegar
- Spring mix or other tender lettuce
- Golden raisins
- Sliced red onion
- Chopped toasted cashews

- Cilantro leaves

Instructions

1. Fill 1/4 of the smoker box with hickory wood chips, and preheat to 225°F. Season chicken thighs all over with salt and pepper. Place thighs directly on the top rack of the smoker. Smoke for about 2 hours or until the internal temperature reaches 165°F. Let rest for 5 minutes. Remove the chicken skin, and pull the chicken into bite-sized pieces. Set aside.

2. While the chicken is cooking, prepare the vinaigrette. Warm 1 tablespoon olive oil in a large skillet over medium heat. Add the onion, garlic, ginger and a pinch of salt, and cook, stirring occasionally, until soft (about 5 minutes). Add the spices, and cook, stirring frequently, for 1 minute. Transfer aromatics to a blender with vinegar, and blend until smooth. With the blender running, add 2/3 cup olive oil in a slow stream to form the vinaigrette. Season to taste with salt.

3. Place pulled chicken in a medium bowl, and add several spoonfuls of the vinaigrette. Toss to combine. The chicken should be well-coated in the sauce, but not drowning in it. Season to taste with additional salt.

4. To serve, place a handful of salad greens on a plate. Place 1/4 of the chicken salad on top of the greens. Top with a sprinkling of raisins, red onion, cashews and cilantro leaves. Finish with a drizzle of vinaigrette. Serve additional vinaigrette on the side.

15. Tomato and Lentil Salad with Feta Cheese and Herbs

Prep Time: 00 Minutes

Cook Time: 15 Minutes

Servings: 4

Ingredients

- 1 torpedo onion, trimmed and thinly sliced (or use a small red onion or two shallots)
- 1 1/2 tablespoons red wine vinegar
- Kosher salt
- 1 1/4 cups whole green lentils
- 3 tablespoons olive oil
- 1 garlic clove, grated or minced
- Freshly ground black pepper
- 3 tablespoons chopped chives, plus more for sprinkling
- 3 tablespoons chopped dill, plus more for sprinkling
- 3 tablespoons chopped Italian parsley, plus more for sprinkling
- 1/2 pound 8 ounces, cherry tomatoes, halved or quartered if large
- 3 ounces feta cheese, crumbled
- Flaky sea salt, for sprinkling

Instructions

1. Add onion in a medium bowl, and toss with vinegar and a pinch of kosher salt. Let sit while you prepare the lentils.

2. Place lentils in a medium saucepan filled 2/3's with water, and bring to a boil over medium-high heat, stirring occasionally. Reduce heat to medium-low, and simmer until the lentils are just tender (about 15 minutes). Start checking for doneness around 13 to 14 minutes, because if you overcook the lentils, they will turn to mush.

3. Drain the lentils well, then toss with the marinated onion. Stir in olive oil and garlic, and season to taste with salt and pepper. Let lentils cool completely.

4. Add chopped herbs to the bowl along with half of the tomatoes and feta, tossing to combine. Pour salad onto a serving platter, then top with remaining tomatoes and feta. Finish with a sprinkling of herbs, flaky sea salt and ground black pepper.

16. Tomato and Watermelon Gazpacho

Prep Time: 00 Minutes

Cook Time: 15 Minutes

Servings: 6

Ingredients

For the gazpacho:

- 4 1/4 pounds whole peeled tomatoes (from 4 28-ounce cans)
- 2 2/3 cups seeded and diced watermelon
- 6 celery stalks, trimmed and finely chopped
- 1 small onion, peeled and finely chopped
- 5 garlic cloves, chopped
- 2 1/2 slices (3 1/2 ounces) french bread, cubed
- 2/3 cup canned tomato puree
- 1/2 cup basil leaves
- 2 tablespoons red wine vinegar
- Scant 1 cup olive oil
- Kosher salt
- Freshly ground black pepper

For the croutons:

- 4 slices 5 ounces french bread, torn into bite-sized pieces
- 3 tablespoons olive oil
- Kosher salt
- To finish: small basil leaves, extra virgin olive oil, flaky sea salt

Instructions

1. Start by preparing the soup. Working in batches if needed, place tomatoes, watermelon, celery, onion, garlic, bread, tomato puree, basil, 1 teaspoon salt and several turns of black pepper in a blender, and blend just until smooth. With the blender going, stream in the vinegar and olive oil. Transfer to a large bowl, and store covered in the fridge until ready to serve.

2. To make the croutons, preheat and oven to 400°F. Add bread to a medium bowl, and toss with olive oil and a few pinches of salt. Transfer to a baking sheet, and cook, tossing occasionally, until crispy and golden (about 15 minutes). Let cool completely.

3. Just before serving, season gazpacho to taste with additional salt and pepper. To serve, ladle soup into

bowls, then top with croutons, basil leaves, a drizzle of extra virgin olive oil and a sprinkling of flaky sea salt.

17. White Bean Risotto with Garlicky Greens

Prep Time: 10 Minutes

Cook Time: 60 Minutes

Servings: 4

Ingredients

- 1/2 cup extra-virgin olive oil
- 3 cloves garlic
- 5 cups low-sodium chicken stock
- 2 tablespoons garlic oil
- 1 medium yellow onion, chopped
- 1/4 teaspoon fresh thyme leaves
- Kosher salt
- 1/2 cup DaVinci Pinot Grigio
- 1 cup risotto rice (I used carnaroli rice)
- 1 cup cooked white beans (I used canned cannellini beans)
- 1/2 cup grated Parmesan cheese, plus more for sprinkling
- 2 tablespoons unsalted butter
- Freshly ground black pepper

- 2 bunches (1 3/4 pounds) bitter greens (I used kale and swiss chard), stems removed and chopped

Instructions

1. Warm 1/2 cup olive oil and garlic in a small saucepan over medium-low heat. Cook until the garlic starts to brown (8 – 10 minutes). Strain oil into a clean container, and discard solids.
2. Bring chicken stock to a simmer in a medium saucepan over medium heat. Once simmering, reduce heat to low, and keep warm.
3. In a large, heavy-bottom pot, warm 2 tablespoons of the garlic oil made in step 1 over medium heat. Add the onion and thyme along with a pinch of salt, and cook until the onion is tender but not browned (6 minutes). Stir in the rice and cook for 2 minutes, then add the Pinot Grigio and cook for 1 more minute. Add 1 cup of warm chicken stock and a pinch of salt, and cook, stirring occasionally, until all of the liquid has been absorbed. Continue adding warm chicken stock 1/2 cup at a time, waiting until the stock is absorbed before adding again, and stirring frequently to make sure the bottom doesn't burn. Continue until the rice is cooked

through, but still al dente, about 30 - 35 minutes total. You may not use all of the chicken stock. Stir in the beans and cook until heated through (1 - 2 minutes). Take the risotto off the heat, and stir in Parmesan cheese and butter. Season to taste with salt and black pepper.

4. During the last 5 minutes of cooking, fill a large pot with an inch or two of water. Place a vegetable steamer on the bottom of the pot, then bring the water to a boil over high heat. Add the chopped greens to the steamer, cover and cook for 5 minutes. Transfer greens to a medium bowl, and drizzle with garlic oil (from step 1), and season to taste with salt and black pepper.

18. Hard-Boiled Egg Toast with Harissa Butter

Prep Time: 5 Minutes

Cook Time: 00 Minutes

Servings: 1

Ingredients

- 2 tablespoons softened, unsalted butter
- 1 teaspoon Harissa, homemade or store-bought
- Kosher salt
- Freshly squeezed lemon juice
- 1 3/4-inch thick slice of bread (multigrain used here)
- 1 hard-boiled egg, sliced (check out my Foolproof Hard-Boiled Eggs)
- Parsley leaves
- Freshly ground black pepper

Instructions

1. Add butter and harissa to a small bowl, stirring to combine. Season to taste with kosher salt and a squeeze of lemon juice. This makes enough Harissa Butter for 2 slices of toast. Set aside.

2. Preheat an oven to 450°F. Toast bread in the oven until lightly golden (about 5 minutes). Spread half of the Harissa Butter on the toast, then top with sliced hard-boiled egg and several small parsley leaves. Season to taste with kosher salt, freshly ground black pepper and a squeeze of lemon juice. Store any unused Harissa Butter in the refrigerator for up to 2 weeks.

19. Gingham's Fried Brussels sprouts

Prep Time: oo Minutes

Cook Time: 2 Minutes

Servings: 6

Ingredients

For the dressing:

- 1 cup apple cider vinegar
- 1/2 cup honey
- 2 salt-packed anchovies, rinsed and minced
- 1 cup jalapeño chiles, seeded and minced
- 1/2 cup fresh garlic, minced
- Kosher salt and freshly ground black pepper, to taste

For the sprouts:

- Canola oil, for frying
- 2 pounds brussels sprouts, stems trimmed and cut in half

Finishing touches:

- 1/2 cup smoked almonds, crushed
- Kosher salt, to taste

Instructions

1. Make the dressing: In a medium bowl, whisk together all the dressing ingredients until smooth. Set aside.

2. Cook the brussels: In a large pan, heat oil to very hot (near smoking) and fry the brussels until crispy, about 1 to 2 minutes. (BE CAREFUL. They will pop! A splatter screen is strongly recommended.)

3. Drain the the brussels sprouts on paper towels, then toss them with the dressing, smoked almonds, and salt to taste.

20. Zucchini Pizza

Prep Time: 30 Minutes

Cook Time: 00 Minutes

Servings: 1

Ingredients

- 1 zucchini (9 ounces), ends trimmed
- 3 garlic cloves, 1 grated or minced, 2 thinly sliced
- Kosher salt
- Olive oil
- 1 ball pizza dough
- 8 ounces mozzarella cheese
- 1/2 small lemon, halved, thinly sliced, seeds removed
- 4 ounces goat cheese, crumbled
- 1 1/2 tablespoons thinly sliced chives

Instructions

1. Cut zucchini in half lengthwise, then cut each half into half-moons. In a medium bowl, toss zucchini with 1 clove grated or minced garlic and 3/4 teaspoon kosher salt. Transfer zucchini to a mesh strainer and set over

the bowl. Let drain for 30 minutes, tossing occasionally. Place zucchini in the middle of a double layer of paper towels. Bring the paper towels up around the zucchini, and gently squeeze to release excess moisture. Pat zucchini dry and set aside.

2. Preheat an oven to 500°F, and set an oven rack in the lowest possible position. Lightly coat a pizza pan with nonstick cooking spray.

3. Stretch pizza dough into a round large enough to fit the pizza pan. Very lightly drizzle the dough with olive oil, using your hands to evenly spread the oil around. Sprinkle dough with a small pinch of kosher salt. Top pizza evenly with grated mozzarella cheese, then evenly scatter 2 thinly sliced garlic cloves, prepared zucchini, lemon pieces and goat cheese over top. Sprinkle the surface of the pizza with a little kosher salt and then lightly drizzle with olive oil.

4. Transfer pizza to the oven on the lowest rack and cook until the crust is golden brown (bottom and crust) and the cheese is nice and bubbly (9 - 11 minutes). Finish the pizza with a sprinkling of chives.

DINNER

21. Corned Beef and Cabbage

Prep Time: 10 Minutes

Cook Time: 8hrs 2 Minutes

Servings: 6

Ingredients

Corned Beef and Cabbage

- 3-4 lb corned beef brisket, plus seasoning packet
- 2 large yellow onions, quartered
- 4 garlic cloves minced
- 2 bay leaves
- ¼ teaspoon whole cloves (about 4 whole cloves) or a pinch of ground clove
- ½ teaspoon dried oregano
- 1 teaspoon black pepper
- 12 ounces beer (any kind will work)
- 1 cup water
- 2 tablespoons apple cider vinegar (or red wine vinegar)
- 1 lb baby potatoes (if using regular potatoes, cut into quarters)

- 1 lb carrots, peeled and cut into 2 "chunks

Fried Cabbage

- 1 head green cabbage, core removed and cut into 1" pieces
- ¼ cup olive oil
- 2 garlic cloves, minced
- Salt, to taste
- Pepper, to taste
- ¼ tsp crushed red pepper flakes, optional

Instructions

Crock Pot Corned Beef Dinner

1. Trim corned beef of excess fat. Rinse under cold water for 1-2 minutes to rinse off excess salt.
2. Place onions, garlic, potatoes and carrots in the bottom of your slow cooker. Add corned beef brisket on top of vegetables, fat side facing up.
3. Add seasoning packet, bay leaves, cloves, oregano, black pepper, beer, water and vinegar. Stir gently to combine.

4. Cook on low for 8-10 hours or until beef is tender and falls apart with your fork.

5. Remove corned beef from crockpot and place on a serving tray. Slice against the grain and serve with vegetables and extra juice.

Instant Pot Corned Beef Dinner

1. Trim corned beef of excess fat. Rinse under cold water for 1-2 minutes to rinse off excess salt.

2. Place onions and garlic in bottom of instant pot. Place corned beef brisket on top.

3. Add seasoning packet, bay leaves, cloves, oregano, black pepper, beer, water and vinegar. Stir gently to combine.

4. Cover, and set instant pot to pressure cook on high for 1 hour and 25 minutes.

5. Let pressure naturally release for 10 minutes, then use the quick release for remaining pressure.

6. Open lid, flip corned beef over and remove about 2 cups of liquid with a ladle (set liquid aside).

7. Add potatoes and carrots to instant pot. Cover and set to pressure cook on high for 5 minutes. Use the quick release to release pressure.

8. Remove corned beef and vegetables from instant pot and serve.

22. Roasted Butternut Squash Feta Pasta

Prep Time: 10 Minutes

Cook Time: 40 Minutes

Servings: 6

Ingredients

- 6 cups butternut squash, cut into 1" cubes (about 1 large squash)
- 8 ounces block Feta cheese
- 1 head of garlic, top 1" cut off
- ⅓-1/2 cup olive oil
- 1 teaspoon salt
- ½ teaspoon pepper
- 1 teaspoon fresh rosemary, chopped
- 1 tablespoon fresh sage, chopped
- ¼ teaspoon ground nutmeg
- 4 cups pasta (I used cavatappi)

Instructions

1. Preheat oven to 425 F. Place cubed butternut squash in large roasting pan. Drizzle generously with olive oil

(about ¼ cup). Season with salt, pepper, rosemary, sage and nutmeg. Toss to evenly combine.

2. Add the block of feta to the middle of the baking dish. Drizzle both sides with olive oil. Place the head of garlic in a piece of aluminum or parchment paper. Drizzle with olive oil. Seal the foil (or if using parchment paper with kitchen twine) and place in baking dish.

3. Bake for 35-40 minutes or until the squash is tender and slightly browned and the feta is soft.

4. Meanwhile, cook pasta in salted water according to package directions to "al dente". Reserve about 1 cup of the pasta water before you drain it. Drizzle pasta with olive oil to prevent sticking and set aside.

5. Once butternut squash and feta are done, remove the pan from the oven and set the garlic aside. Immediately stir the feta and squash together (the feta should be creamy). Add the cooked pasta and stir.

6. Squeeze out the roasted garlic into the pasta and stir to combine. Add pasta water as needed if pasta is too dry.

7. Season with salt and pepper and serve.

23. Thai Chicken Rice Bowls with Peanut Sauce

Prep Time: 30 Minutes

Cook Time: 15 Minutes

Servings: 4

Ingredients

Thai Chicken Marinade:

- 1.5-2lbs boneless, skinless chicken thighs
- ½ cup coconut milk
- 2 tablespoons lime juice, about 1 lime
- 2 tablespoons fish sauce
- 3 tablespoons brown sugar (or honey)
- 1 tablespoon avocado or olive oil
- 1 tablespoon green curry paste

Peanut Sauce:

- ½ cup creamy peanut butter
- 2 tablespoons soy sauce
- 2 tablespoons brown sugar (or honey)
- 1 tablespoon lime juice (about ½ lime)
- 1 teaspoon minced garlic (about 2 cloves)
- 2 teaspoons grated ginger

- ¼ cup coconut milk (plus more as needed to thin out)

Rice Bowls:

- 4 cups cooked rice such as jasmine, white or brown rice
- 1 large head of broccoli
- Olive oil, for roasting
- Salt and pepper, to taste
- 1 large cucumber, diced
- 2 carrots, shredded into ribbons
- Bunch of scallions, sliced, for serving
- 1 cup crushed peanuts, for serving
- Bunch of fresh herbs such as cilantro, mint and/or basil, for serving

Instructions

1. For the Thai chicken: combine all marinade ingredients in a small bowl. Place chicken thighs in zip lock bag or large bowl. Pour marinade over the chicken and massage to evenly coat. Cover or seal and refrigerate for at least 2 hours or up to 24 hours.

2. Make the peanut sauce: combine all peanut sauce ingredients in a large glass jar or bowl. Whisk or shake to evenly combine (I like to microwave it for about 30 seconds so it's easier to mix together). Add additional coconut milk as needed until desired consistency. Store peanut sauce in jar or air tight container in refrigerator up to 1 week.

3. Roast the broccoli: spread broccoli florets evenly on to a baking sheet (or you can do this on the grill). Drizzle with a little olive oil and sprinkle with salt and pepper. Roast 20-25 minutes until browned, set aside.

4. Prepare rice according to package directions and set aside.

5. Remove chicken from refrigerator 30 mins prior to grilling to let it come to room temp (this allows it to cook evenly). Preheat grill on medium-high heat. Spray with nonstick cooking spray and add chicken. Cook 3-5 minutes per side until you have nice grill

marks and the chicken is fully cooked through. Remove and set aside.

6. Assemble your rice bowls: add about 1 cup of rice to each bowl. Top with roasted broccoli, diced cucumbers, carrots, green onions, peanuts and herbs. Top each bowl with a piece of the grilled chicken and drizzle with a generous amount of peanut sauce.

7. Serve and enjoy!

24. Butternut Squash Pasta Bake with Sausage

Prep Time: 35 Minutes

Cook Time: 35 Minutes

Servings: 8

Ingredients

For The Roasted Butternut Squash:

- 3 cups butternut squash, peeled and cubed
- Olive oil, for drizzling
- 1 teaspoon ground nutmeg
- Pinch of salt
- Pinch of black pepper

For The Pasta Bake:

- 1 lb pasta (I used rigatoni)
- 2 tablespoons olive oil
- ½ cup onion, diced (about 1 small onion)
- 1 lb ground Italian sausage (mild or hot)
- 1 tablespoon garlic, minced (about 3 cloves)
- 4 cups kale, thick stems removed and roughly chopped
- 16 ounces ricotta cheese
- 4 ounces goat cheese, crumbled

- 1 cup shredded mozzarella cheese, divided
- ½ cup freshly grated Parmesan cheese
- ¾ cup milk
- 1 tablespoon fresh sage (or 2 teaspoons ground sage)
- ¼ teaspoon ground nutmeg
- 1 tablespoon Dijon mustard
- ½ teaspoon kosher salt
- ½ teaspoon black pepper

Instructions

1. Roast the butternut squash: preheat oven to 425 F. Place cubed squash on large baking sheet. Drizzle with olive oil and sprinkle with 1 teaspoon nutmeg, salt and pepper. Bake 20-25 minutes, stirring halfway, or until squash is tender and slightly caramelized. Remove and set aside.

2. While the butternut squash is roasting, cook the pasta in a large pot of salted water according to package directions to "al-dente". Drain and drizzle with olive oil to prevent sticking. Set aside.

3. When squash is done cooking, turn oven down to 375 F. Spray a 13" x 9" baking dish lightly with cooking spray, set aside.

4. In a large sauté pan, heat olive oil over medium-high heat. Add onion, cook 2 minutes then add ground sausage. Cook until sausage is no longer pink and lightly browned, using wooden spoon to crumble it. Stir in garlic and cook 1 minute.

5. Add kale, turn off heat, cover and cook until kale is wilted.

6. Meanwhile, in a medium bowl combine: ricotta, goat cheese, ½ cup mozzarella, Parmesan, milk, sage, ground nutmeg, Dijon, salt and pepper.

7. In a large bowl (or the same pan you cooked pasta), combine butternut squash, cooked pasta, kale and sausage mixture and cheese mixture. Stir to combine.

8. Spread into 13" x 9" baking dish. Top with remaining ½ cup of mozzarella cheese. Cover with foil and bake 20 minutes, then remove foil and bake for additional 15-20 minutes or until cheese is melted and mixture is bubbling.

25. Honey Mustard Roasted Pork Tenderloin

Prep Time: 15 Minutes

Cook Time: 45 Minutes

Servings: 4

Ingredients

For The Dry Rub:

- 1 lb pork tenderloin
- 1 tablespoon olive oil
- 1 teaspoon garlic powder
- ½ teaspoon onion powder
- 1 teaspoon dried rosemary (or 1 tablespoon fresh)
- ½ teaspoon dried thyme (or 1.5 teaspoons fresh)
- ½ teaspoon smoked paprika
- 1 teaspoon kosher salt
- ½ teaspoon black pepper

For The Honey Mustard Glaze:

- 2 tablespoons honey
- ¼ cup whole grain mustard
- ½ teaspoon dried rosemary (or 1.5 teaspoons fresh)
- 1 tablespoon apple cider vinegar

- 1 tablespoon brown sugar

- Pinch of salt

For The Vegetables:

- 2 yellow onions, peeled and cut into quarters

- 4 carrots, peeled

- 2 cups potatoes, quartered (I like the baby potatoes)

- 1 whole head of garlic, top trimmed

- ¼ cup olive oil

Instructions

1. Coat pork tenderloin with olive oil. In a small bowl combine remaining dry rub ingredients: garlic and onion powder, rosemary, thyme, smoked paprika, salt and pepper. Generously rub all over the pork tenderloin. Set aside.

2. In another small bowl, combine all ingredients for the honey mustard glaze, set aside.

3. Preheat the oven to 425 F. In a large cast iron skillet (or other oven safe skillet), add onions, carrots, potatoes and garlic. Drizzle generously with olive oil (about ¼ cup). Season with salt and pepper. Roast in the oven for 20 minutes.

4. Remove from oven and place skillet on stove top over medium-high heat. Turn oven down to 400 F. Push vegetables aside and add pork, searing for 2-3 minutes per side until golden brown. (I like to give the vegetables a stir at this time too).

5. Brush pork with half of the honey mustard glaze. Place skillet back into the oven and cook for 10 minutes. Remove from oven, flip pork over and brush with remaining honey mustard glaze. Roast again for additional 10 minutes or until the internal temperature reaches 145 F.

6. Remove skillet from oven and place pork on cutting board. Let rest at least 5 minutes before slicing and serving.

26. Ground Turkey & Broccoli Noodle Casserole

Prep Time: 25 Minutes

Cook Time: 25 Minutes

Servings: 6

Ingredients

- 2 cups whole wheat egg noodles
- 2 tablespoons olive oil, divided, plus more for drizzling the top
- 1 lb lean ground turkey (can substitute with ground chicken or shredded chicken breast)
- 2 cups broccoli, cut into small florets
- 1 cup carrots, thinly sliced
- Salt
- Pepper
- 1 tablespoon (3 cloves) garlic, minced
- 1 tablespoon butter
- ½ cup yellow onion, diced
- 3 tablespoons flour
- 1 ¾ cup chicken broth
- 1 cup milk
- 1 ½ teaspoons fresh thyme (or ½ teaspoon dried)

- ½ cup shredded mozzarella cheese
- 4 ounces cream cheese, softened and cubed
- 3 tablespoons panko (or regular bread crumbs)
- 1 tablespoon grated Parmesan cheese

Instructions

1. Preheat oven to 375 degrees. Spray a 13 x 9 baking dish with cooking spray. Set aside.
2. Cook noodles in salted water according to package directions to al dente or undercook by 2 minutes. Drain, toss with olive oil to avoid sticking, and set aside.
3. Meanwhile, in a large sauté pan, heat 1 tablespoon olive oil over medium heat. Add ground turkey and cook 5-7 minutes until no longer pink and slightly browned. Remove from pan and set aside in a large bowl.
4. Return pan to stove, add remaining 1 tablespoon olive oil. Add broccoli, carrots, pinch of salt and pepper. Cover, and cook 2-3 minutes until softened. Remove cover, add garlic and cook 1 minute. Remove from pan and set aside in the bowl with the ground turkey.
5. Return pan to stave again. Add butter. Once melted, add onions and cook about 5 minutes until translucent

and softened. Add flour, cook 1 minute. Slowly whisk in broth, adding a little at a time, then add the milk and thyme.

6. Bring mixture to a boil, then lower and simmer 5-7 minutes until slightly thickened (it should coat the back of the spoon).

7. Stir in mozzarella and cream cheese. Remove from heat.

8. Add back the ground turkey, broccoli and carrots. Then stir in the egg noodles.

9. Pour mixture in 13x9 casserole dish. Top with panko and grated cheese, drizzle with olive oil. Bake for 20-25 minutes or until the top is lightly browned and cheeses are bubbling.

27. Asian Air Fryer Salmon

Prep Time: 30 Minutes

Cook Time: 10 Minutes

Servings: 4

Ingredients

- 4 salmon fillets, about 6 ounces each
- 1 tablespoon olive oil
- 1 teaspoon fresh ginger, grated
- 1 tablespoon brown sugar, or honey
- 1 teaspoon garlic, minced
- 2 tablespoons soy sauce (light sodium preferred)
- 2 tablespoons lime juice (about 1 lime)
- ¼ cup sweet chili sauce, for glazing

Instructions

1. Combine olive oil, ginger, brown sugar, garlic, soy sauce and lime juice in a small bowl.
2. Place salmon in zip lock back. Pour marinade on top and gently massage to evenly coat the salmon. Place in refrigerator for at least 30 minutes or up to a day.

3. Once salmon has marinated, preheat your air fryer for 5 minutes at 380 F.

4. Place salmon pieces onto hot air fryer basket, skin side down. Close and set your air fryer to 380 F for 5 minutes.

5. Remove basket and brush each piece of salmon with sweet chili glaze. Place back into air fryer and cook an additional 2-3 minutes or until desired doneness is reached.

6. Serve and enjoy!

28. Chai Pumpkin Cheesecake with Salted Caramel

Prep Time: 20 Minutes

Cook Time: 1hr 10 Minutes

Servings: 12

Ingredients

For The Gingersnap Crust:

- 14 ounces gingersnap cookie crumbs (about 2. 5 cups)
- 1 tablespoon brown sugar
- ½ cup (1 stick) unsalted butter, melted

For The Cheesecake Filling:

- 2 pounds (4 packages) cream cheese, room temperature
- 1 cup granulated sugar
- ¾ cup brown sugar
- ½ teaspoon salt
- 5 large eggs, room temperature
- 2 tablespoons all-purpose flour
- 1 cup pumpkin purée (not pumpkin pie mix)
- ¾ cup sour cream, room temperature
- 2 teaspoons vanilla extract

- 2 tablespoons chai spice

For Whipped Cream Topping (Optional):

- ½ cup heavy cream

- 1 teaspoon vanilla extract

- 1 tablespoon granulated sugar

- 1 teaspoon chai spice

Salted Caramel Drizzle

- Homemade salted caramel sauce,

Instructions

Make The Gingersnap Crust:

1. Preheat oven to 350 F. Add gingersnap cookie crumbs and brown sugar to a large mixing bowl. Stir in the melted butter and mix until evenly combined.

2. Transfer mixture to bottom of a 9 or 10 "springform pan. Using your hands (or bottom of a glass), press crust firmly into bottom and about halfway up the sides of the pan.

3. Bake for 12-15 minutes until lightly golden and fragrant. Remove from oven let cool while you make the filling.

Make The Filling:

1. Reduce oven temperature to 300 F. In stand mixer with paddle attachment (or with a hand beater), beat room temp cream cheese, sugars and salt until smooth and creamy (about 2-3 minutes).
2. Scrape down the bowl as needed. Add in the eggs, one at a time, and beating after each addition just until blended.
3. Add flour, pumpkin puree, sour cream, chai spices and vanilla. Scrape down sides and bottom of bowl and mix just until combined.

Prepare Water Bath & Bake:

1. Fill tea kettle or medium pot with water and bring to a boil. While water is heating up, wrap bottom and sides of springform pan tightly in aluminum foil, about halfway up the pan (this is to prevent the water from leaking into the pan).
2. Pour cheesecake filling on top of the prepared gingersnap crust.
3. Place cheesecake in the bottom of a large roasting pan. Carefully pour hot water inside of the roasting pan until it reaches about 1" up the sides of the cheesecake (be careful not to go past the aluminum foil!).

4. Carefully transfer pan to oven. Bake for one hour or until cheesecake is set but center is still wobbly. Shut oven off and let cheesecake sit in the oven for an additional hour (don't open the oven door!).

5. Remove from oven and water bath and let cool to room temperature. Cover and refrigerate for at least 6 hours or overnight.

29. Shrimp Pasta with Cherry Tomatoes, Rosé & Spinach

Prep Time: 15 Minutes

Cook Time: 15 Minutes

Servings: 4

Ingredients

- 1 lb linguine pasta (or other pasta)
- ¼ cup olive oil
- ½ cup yellow onion, diced
- 20 ounces cherry tomatoes (about 3 cups)
- 6 garlic cloves, minced
- Pinch red pepper flakes, optional
- 1 teaspoon salt
- 1 teaspoon black pepper
- 1 lb raw shrimp, peeled and deveined
- ¾ cup dry rosé wine, see recipe notes
- 3 cups baby spinach
- ¼ cup fresh basil, roughly chopped
- 2 tablespoons fresh parsley, chopped
- 1 tablespoon lemon juice (about ½ lemon)
- ⅓ Cup grated Parmesan cheese
- 4 tablespoons butter

Instructions

1. Cook pasta "al dente" according to package directions. Drain and toss with olive oil to prevent sticking. Set aside.
2. Meanwhile, in a large sauté pan, heat olive oil over medium-high heat. Add onions and tomatoes. Cook 5 minutes, stirring occasionally, just until the tomatoes burst and start to lose their shape.
3. Stir in garlic and red pepper flakes (if using). Cook 30 seconds just until garlic is fragrant.
4. Add shrimp, salt and pepper. Reduce heat to medium. Cook shrimp about 2-3 minutes per side or until pink.
5. Stir in wine and cook for 2 minutes. Then add spinach, parsley, and basil and lemon juice and cook until spinach is wilted. Remove from heat.
6. Toss tomato mixture over cooked pasta with butter and Parmesan cheese. Season with salt and pepper if needed.
7. Serve with extra lemon, parsley and cheese if desired.

30. Cardamom Apple Pear Crisp

Prep Time: 20 Minutes

Cook Time: 45 Minutes

Servings: 10

Ingredients

Apple Pear Filling

- 4 pears, peeled & sliced (about 4-5 cups)
- 3 medium-large apples, peeled and sliced (about 4-5 cups)
- ½ cup brown sugar, packed
- ¼ cup all-purpose flour
- 1 teaspoon ground cinnamon
- 1 ½ teaspoon ground cardamom
- ½ teaspoon ground nutmeg
- 1 teaspoon vanilla extract
- 1 tablespoon lemon juice
- ¼ teaspoon kosher salt

Gingersnap Oat Topping

- ¾ cup all-purpose flour
- ⅓ Cup brown sugar

- 1 teaspoon cinnamon
- ¼ teaspoon kosher salt
- 1 stick cold unsalted butter, cubed
- ¾ cup gingersnap cookie crumbs
- ¼ cup old-fashioned oats
- ½ cup pecans, chopped (optional)

Instructions

1. Preheat oven to 350 F. Lightly spray or grease a 9 x 13 inch baking dish or other 3 quart baking dish.
2. In a large bowl mix together all of the filling ingredients: pears, apples, brown sugar, flour, spices, vanilla, lemon juice and salt. Spread evenly into your baking dish.
3. For the topping: In a medium bowl whisk together flour, brown sugar, cinnamon and salt. Cut in the cold butter with either a pastry cutter, two forks or with your hands. The mixture should resemble pea-sized crumbs. Stir in the gingersnap crumbs, oats and nuts (if using).

4. Evenly spread topping on top of pear-apple mixture.

5. Bake for 40-50 minutes or until the top is golden brown and the juices inside are bubbling. Remove and let cool at least 5 minutes before serving.

6. Serve warm or room temperature with vanilla ice cream or whipped cream, if desired.